How To Use
ESSENTIAL OILS

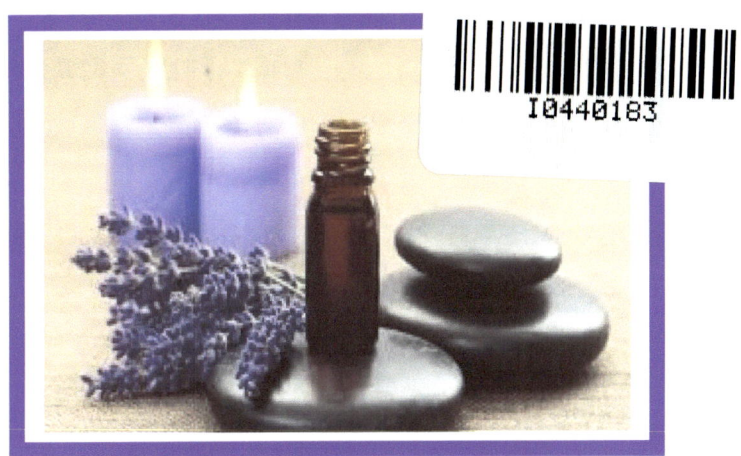

I0440183

Written By:

Dr. Kathleen B. Oden
Certified Health Minister

Create Anewu Health Ministry

Create Anewu Health Ministry©

HOW TO USE ESSENTIAL OILS

For
Health & Wellness

Most essential oils are very potent.

There are 3 ways to use essential oils:

1. **Orally**
2. **Topically**
3. **Inhale**

WARNING!
Never ingest (orally) more than 5-6 drops of essential oil!

Orally

To get the best benefit for health,
3 drops of therapeutic essential oil
should be used. However, more can be
used if you are creating or following,
a recipe.

Topically

Most essential oils should be mixed
with coconut oil, olive oil, or jojoba oil,
before using topically
on face or body.
Mix oils according to recipe.

Inhale

Some, essential oils can be inhaled
directly from the bottle. But it is safer
to use an oil lamp or diffuser.

Weight Loss

When it comes to losing weight, some people know that a healthy diet and doing the right type of exercise, can help with weight loss.

But oftentimes, people want or need an extra boost to help them reach their weight loss goal.

Unfortunately, most people turn to artificial stimulants, like caffeine for weight loss, rather than plant-based medicine.

More Natural Health doctors and health coaches, are now available to help people improve or maintain their health.

Grapefruit essential oil is great to use for weight loss!

Four essential oils that have been proven to support weight loss:

• **GRAPEFRUIT OIL** contains d-limonene, which is found in citrus peels. A study found that supplementing d-limonene improved metabolic enzyme levels.

• **PEPPERMINT OIL** has been shown to improve weight loss because it suppresses cravings and improves digestion.

• **CINNAMON OIL** helps balance blood sugar levels, which will assist in weight loss and improve diabetes.

• **GINGER OIL** contains gingerol, which has powerful anti-inflammatory properties, and increases thermogenesis, which boosts metabolism.

ANTI-AGING & WRINKLE FIGHTER

Frankincense essential oil
is a powerful astringent,
meaning it helps protect skin cells.

It can be used to help
Reduce acne blemishes
and the appearance of large pores,
prevent wrinkles,
and it will even help lift and tighten
skin to naturally slow signs of aging.

Frankincense essential oil
can be used anywhere the skin
becomes saggy,
such as the abdomen, jowls or under
the eyes. Mix six drops of oil to one
ounce of unscented oil and apply it
directly to the skin.

Be sure to always use on a small area
first to test for possible
allergic reactions.

All Essential Oils

Are Not Therapeutic

The majority of essential oils that are made today, are made for the food and fragrance industry. They are not for consumption.

There are hundreds of compounds (different chemicals) in just one essential oil, but not all oils are used for healing purposes.

The fragrance industry is only interested in how the oil smells.

Therefore, they only use the part of the oil that gives the fragrance and then they discard the rest.

The same goes for the medical field. They use a small part of a plant to create medicine and then add in chemicals which are cheaper to use then essential oils.

And the food industry only wants the parts that taste good. So they remove the parts that taste like mint, peppermint, lemon, cinnamon, ... etc., and use it to flavor recipes.

With Therapeutic Oils, none of the compounds are removed, so that we can experience all of the health benefits, that God put into His therapeutic essential oils.

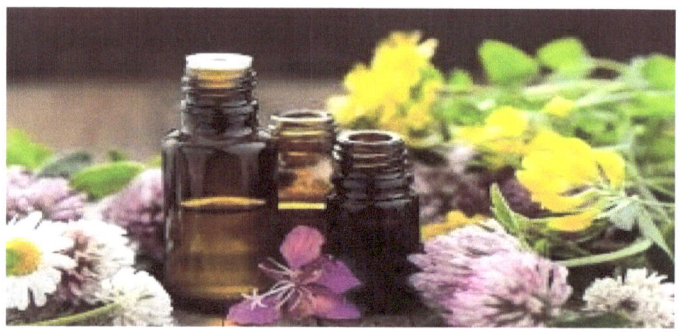

Natural / Organic

Today, we are used to seeing items labeled "natural" or "organic." And we immediately think that item is health food.

The government allows the food industry to use the word "natural" on a product or the word "organic", but that does not mean that it is healthy.

And, today, products can be 100% man-made, and still be labeled as "natural."

100% Pure Therapeutic Essential Oil

Real therapeutic grade essential oils can help to keep your immune system working properly.

Man-made synthetic oils do not. 100% pure essential oils are stored in dark bottles, but synthetic oils come in clear bottles and have no healing compounds in it.

Also, real essential oils cost more.

WHAT ARE ESSENTIAL OILS?

They are mostly extracted by distillation, which separates the oil- and water-based compounds of a plant, by using steam. Essential oils are extracted directly from a plant or tree.

Usually from the bark, flower, fruit, leaf, seed or root. And for most uses, it only takes one drop, because it is so powerful.

The therapeutic oil in plants protects it from the environment and helps plants adapt to their surroundings.

When our bodies absorb essential oils, it is also protected from the environment.

Essential oils are used in many countries, therefore, no one knows where it originated.

They become popular in the United States in the 1980s, when essential oils were added to lotions, candles and other fragrances.

A french chemist first used lavender essential oil in 1928. He discovered that lavender oil could be used for skin infections, wounds and burns.

Today, trained professionals such as doctors of natural medicine, physical therapists, massage therapists and nutritionists use essential oils.

And many hospitals today, are now aware of the benefits of essential oils and are using them in the treatment of anxiety, depression and infections in hospitalized patients.

4 TYPES OF ESSENTIAL OILS

1 - <u>Therapeutic</u> - the best
  - taken straight from the plant

2 - <u>Natural or Organic</u>
- small among of plant compound or
may not contain plant compound...
depends on the company.

3 - <u>Fragrance</u>
- this is an altered oil & contains no
plant compound. Some are man-made.

4 - <u>Synthetic</u>
- totally created in a lab... man-made.

Homemade Hair Conditioner
Total Time: 2 minutes Serves: 20-30

INGREDIENTS:
1 cup water
2 tbsp apple cider vinegar
10 drops of essential oils

Customize Your Conditioner:
Rosemary or sage essential oil

Oils for all types of hair:
Lemon, bergamot, or tea tree
essential oils for oily hair

Lavender, sandalwood or geranium essential
oils for dry hair or dandruff

Use a BPA free plastic bottles or Glass bottle
with dispenser.

DIRECTIONS:
1. Mix ingredients together in 8oz spray bottle
2. Shake bottle before using & then spray hair
3. Leave in hair for 5 minutes then rinse

Pain and Inflammation

USE WINTERGREEN

& PEPPERMINT

Mix with coconut oil

and make a compress.

APPLY FOR 30 SECONDS

ALSO, USE CYPRESS OIL

For inflammation

OR blend all of these together

FOR HEADACHES...
LAVENDER & PEPPERMINT
CYPRESS

Do you need some extra help with weight?

Combine grapefruit oil, ginger oil and cinnamon oil and take as supplement 3x daily to support Metabolism.

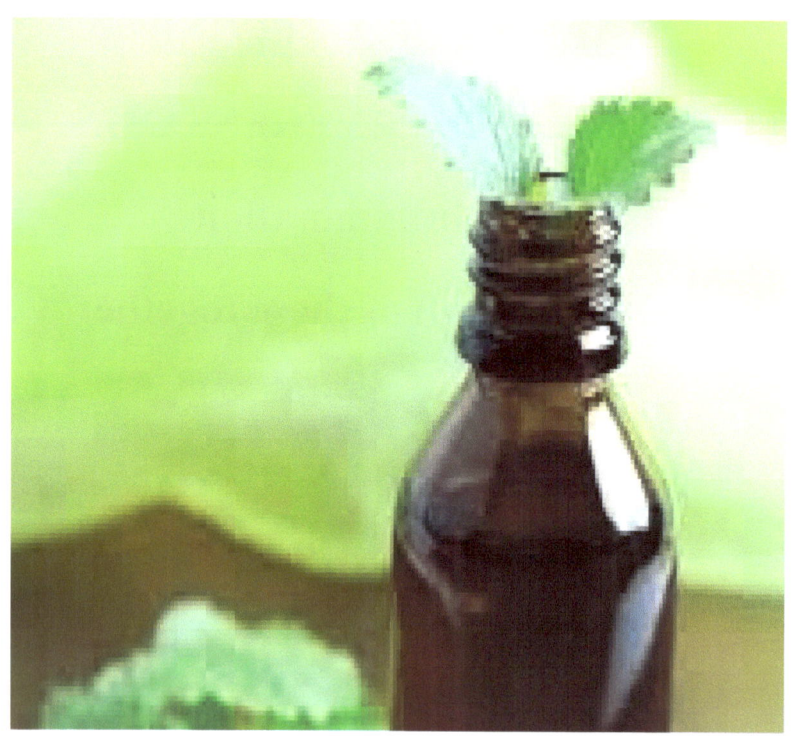

TOP 8 ESSENTIAL OILS TO KEEP ON HAND

FRANKINCENSE - the King of oils...can be used in place of any essential oil. Excellent for any skin condition.

LAVENDER - helps any time you need calming. Excellent for helping you to sleep and for any pain.

PEPPERMENT - helps with any digestive problems like gas or indigestion or a quick pick-me-up, anytime of day.

CINNAMON - helps with weight loss and to balance blood sugar. Excellent oil for people with diabetes.

EUCALYPTUS - helps with all breathing problems like colds, allergies and sinus.

TEA TREE - a natural antibiotic, also speeds up the metabolism for quick weight loss.

OREGANO - kills toenail fungus, athletes foot and yeast infections and also a natural antibiotic

GINGER - helps with nausea, vomiting and indigestion.

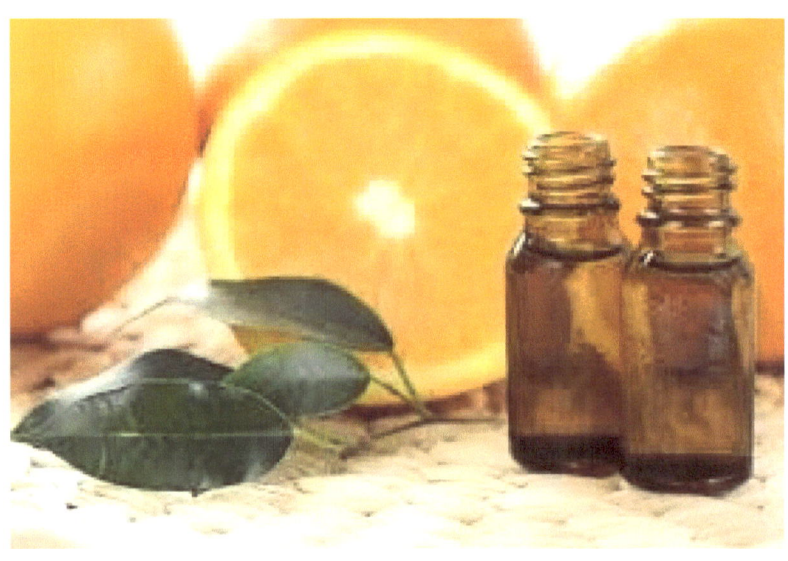

EUCALYPTUS

Eucalyptus essential oil improves respiratory health and fights sinus infections. Also, it decreases mucus production and improves digestive health.

FOR COLDS & FLU

Eucalyptus helps cleanse your body of harmful toxins that can make you feel sick. One of the most effective ways to utilize eucalyptus for colds is to drop 2-3 drops of the essential oil into your diffuser before going to sleep so you can take advantage of the healing benefits all night long.

FOR CUTS, BURNS OR ANTISEPTIC

Eucalyptus is effective at treating wounds, burns, cuts, abrasions, sores and scrapes. Mix with coconut oil to make a salve or healing ointment and put on bug bites and stings. Eucalyptus acts a natural pain reliever and also keeps the area from getting infected.

CINNAMON

Popular Uses of Cinnamon Oil

Place 1 drop Cinnamon essential oil in hot water or tea and drink slowly to soothe your throat.

Put 2–3 drops in a spray bottle for a quick and effective cleaning spray.

Place one drop on your toothbrush then add toothpaste.

Dilute with a carrier oil then apply to cold, achy joints during winter time.

Cooking; cinnamon oil is "Generally Recognized as Safe" (GRAS) by the FDA, and a quality brand may be used in cooking.

Start off with a single drop (or less), until you know your ratios.

FRANKINCENSE

THE KING OF ESSENTIAL OILS

**MAY HELP FIGHT CANCER,
OR DEAL WITH CHEMOTHERAPY
SIDE EFFECTS.**

**Frankincense oil has been shown
to help fight cells of
specific types of cancer.**

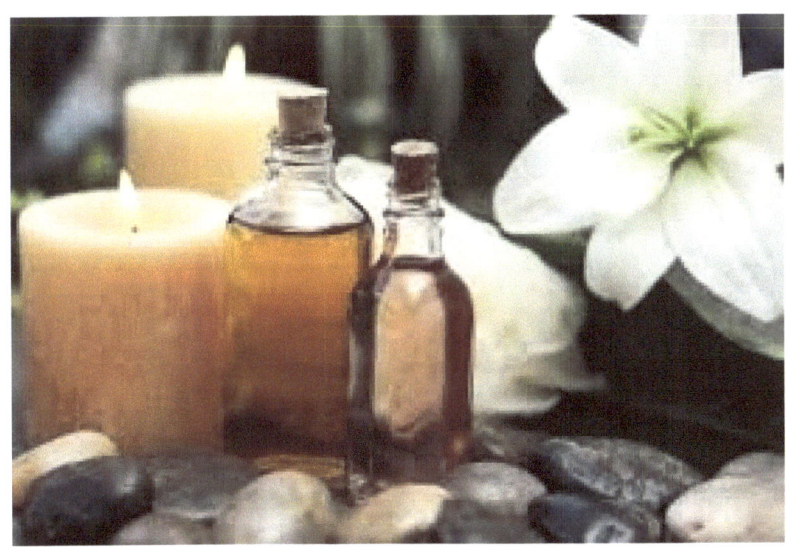

Essential Oils can help our bodies:

Physically, Mentally, Spiritually, and Emotionally

God is the greatest physician ever. He created us, and yet people leave Him out and trust only in "doctors" who most of the time are guessing, at what is going on in our bodies.

God gave us doctors, but He never meant for doctors to replace God.

God created and placed all the food, essential oils, spices and herbs, on earth for our health and healing. We just need to ask God to show us what they are and how to use them.

AMEN!

Cough Syrup

INGREDIENTS:

1 drop of lemon essential oil
1 drop peppermint essential oil
1 drop lavender essential oil
1 spoonful of honey

Put In Glass Jar

DIRECTIONS:

Add the oils with honey.
Mix and consume.

Serves: 1

James 5:14

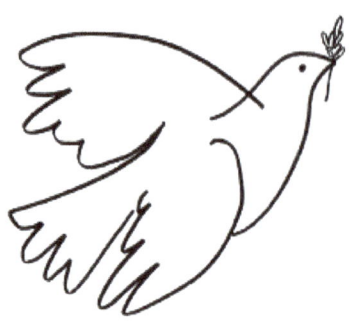

"Is anyone among you sick?

Let him call for the elders

of the church,

and let them pray over him,

anointing him with oil

in the name of the Lord."

Revelation 22:2

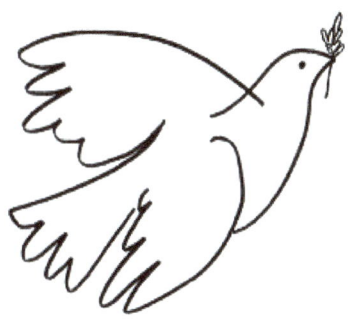

"In the middle of it's street,

and on either side of the river,

was the tree of life,

which bore twelve fruits,

each tree yielding it's fruit every month.

The leaves of the tree were for

the healing of the nations."

Dr. Kathleen B. Oden

Dr. Kathleen B. Oden has been a member of God's House of Refuge Church & School of Evangelism since 1994. She is currently the Church Administrator, Bible teacher and missionary. She graduated from Immanuel Temple, School of the Bible, in 2000, with a Doctorate degree in Christian Theology.

Currently, she has a new ministry called, Create Anewu Health Ministry. She holds healthy eating seminars and she does private health coaching.

Dr. Oden has authored over 15 books through AMAZON.COM and is currently working on several new books.

WEBSITE:
createanewuhealthministry.com

EMAIL:
createanewu@consultant.com